FROM THE HEART *of a* CAREGIVER

WHAT TWENTY YEARS OF CARE TAUGHT ME

GWENDOLYN BURRELL

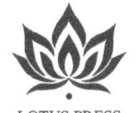

LOTUS PRESS

Lotus Press
Dallas, Texas

Copyright © 2025 by Gwendolyn Burrell.
Published by Lotus Press

Cover Design: mypublishedbook.com
Interior Design by: mypublishedbook.com

All rights reserved. This book or any portion thereof may not be reproduced or used in any manner whatsoever without the express written permission of the publisher except for the use of brief quotations in a book review.

ISBN: 979-8-218-78308-2
Printed in the United States of America.

To my mother, Lydia —

You were my first glimpse of what it means to love and care deeply.

Your gentle spirit, nurturing hands, and quiet strength

shaped the very foundation of who I am.

You didn't just teach me how to care, you lived
it, every day, with grace and kindness.

Thank you for planting the seeds of compassion, for teaching me the value of herbs,

healing, and holistic wisdom, and for showing
me the sacred power of a mother's love.

This book, and the heart behind it, is because of you.

With love always,

Gwendolyn

Contents

Introduction 9
Chapter 1: Rooted in Love — My Personal Story. 11
Chapter 2: When You Begin to Notice the Changes 15
Chapter 3: Helping Them Feel Safe. 19
Chapter 4: The Power of Music & Nature in Healing. 23
Chapter 5: Choosing the Right Caregiver or Companion 27
Chapter 6: When Your Loved One Moves into Assisted Living 31
Chapter 7: When a Caregiver Becomes Family 35
Chapter 8: Selecting an Assisted Living Community or Residential Care Home 39
Chapter 9: The Power of Holistic Healing – Herbs, Oils, Supplements & More. 43
Chapter 10: Tips for Selecting a Caregiver. 47
Chapter 11: A Caregiver's Heart – A Gentle Reminder to Families. . .51
Chapter 12: Alzheimer's and Dementia – Home Health Care & Hope 55
Chapter 13: When the Sun Goes Down – Meeting the Soul at Dusk . 57
Chapter 14: Closing Reflection – The Journey of Love & Care 61
Appendix 63
Care Logs and Journals 63
Acknowledgements 67
About the Author. 71

Introduction

Caregiving is one of the most sacred and challenging journeys a person can take. Whether planned or unexpected, stepping into the role of caregiver changes your life and your heart forever.

This guide was born from over twenty years of hands-on experience caring for elders, including those navigating memory loss, illness, and end-of-life transitions. In these pages you'll find honest reflections, practical advice, and soulful encouragement. From the first signs that something is changing to choosing the right caregiver, creating comforting routines, and embracing holistic tools like music, herbs, and touch, this book offers support for every stage of the caregiving journey.

The chapters are designed to stand alone, so you can read straight through or turn to the section that meets your need in the moment. The appendix includes care logs and journaling pages to help you stay organized and emotionally grounded.

My hope is that this book will be both a companion and a compass, offering gentle guidance, emotional validation, and a reminder that you are not alone. No matter where you are on the path, may you always be rooted in love.

Chapter 1

ROOTED IN LOVE — MY PERSONAL STORY

I had a unique life as a child, one that shaped my heart and path long before I ever realized it. I was raised by older parents, which meant that my world was naturally filled with the rhythms, wisdom, and presence of elders. While many children spent their time running around with peers, I found myself most at ease sitting beside someone decades older than me—listening, learning, and laughing. Older people were not strangers to me, they were my friends, my guides, my companions.

I vividly remember one summer day, swinging on an old porch swing, laughing and talking with a woman in her fifties while I was just ten. She was a neighbor but she was also one of my best friends. Our conversations, though simple, were layered with wisdom I didn't yet know I was gathering. That kind of connection left a lasting imprint on me. It taught me early on that every wrinkle held a story, every slow step carried history, and every elder was a living library.

Nature was also a constant companion in my childhood. Summers were spent outside—barefoot, wide-eyed, and full of imagination. My father, after retiring, was a farmer. He grew all kinds of vegetables and sold them to local markets. He was both tending soil and nurturing life. My twin sister and I would play nearby, surrounded by tall tomato plants, rows of collard greens, corn stalks reaching for the sky, black-eyed pea vines twisting through the garden beds, and vibrant strawberry patches bursting with color. We created magic in those moments. We were at home with nature.

From my mother, I inherited a love for herbs, oils, and holistic healing. She believed in the gentle power of natural remedies and always reached for the most nurturing solution first. Her teachings planted seeds in me that would later grow into a deeper understanding of how mind, body, and spirit connect, especially in the care of others. Her influence helped shape how I care for people and how I view health and healing in a broader, more intuitive way.

My mother was also the true cornerstone of my life. She epitomized grace. With gentle hands and calming words, she had a way of bringing peace even to the most unsettled souls. She was, without question, the love of my life. What she gave to me was kindness, patience, and an understanding heart that I now give to others.

As I grew older, the seeds planted in my childhood, the love for nature, the wisdom of elders, and the care my mother modeled, began to take root in unexpected ways. At first, I followed a different path. I explored business, fashion merchandising, real estate, and even the semiconductor industry. Each stop along the way added something to my understanding of people, professionalism, and life. But something was always calling me to my childhood first loves.

Eventually, that calling led me into the medical field. Becoming a medical assistant felt like returning home. I was helping, healing, and connecting with others, especially the ancestral ways that felt natural and deeply fulfilling. I worked for a visiting physicians' group, and part of my role was to accompany the doctor on home visits. Most of our patients were older adults, and being welcomed into their homes reminded me of my younger years. Sitting and talking with someone much older felt like the most normal thing in the world.

What struck me most was what happened after the visits. These patients still needed help with organizing medications, understanding instructions, or just someone to check in and care. And so, I returned. Not because I was asked, and certainly not for pay, but because my heart compelled me to do so. It was in those moments that I knew I had come full circle. I remembered the swing, the soft voice of my mother, the peace of the garden, and the warmth of human connection.

God was showing me that caring for the elderly one-on-one was my purpose. It had always been there. And even when I wasn't being paid, I was still showing up, still giving, still loving. That's when you know something is more than a job; it's a calling.

Caregiving is not what I do. It's who I am.

Chapter 2

WHEN YOU BEGIN TO NOTICE THE CHANGES

Caring for a loved one doesn't usually begin with a loud alarm or a dramatic event. It often starts quietly. A forgotten appointment. A misplaced purse. A story told twice within the same conversation. These small moments, that are easy to brush off at first, can become more frequent, more noticeable. You may find yourself wondering: Is something going on?

Recognizing these early signs is often the very first step in a family's caregiving journey. And though it can be difficult to face, noticing the changes early allows us to step in with love and prepare for what may lie ahead.

It's natural to feel unsure in the beginning. Many people hesitate to mention what they're seeing because they don't want to embarrass their loved one or themselves. But the most important thing to remember is that noticing a change is not the same as labeling it. It's simply observing with love and care.

Maybe your mother is forgetting to take her medication, or your father's once spotless home is looking neglected. These can be signs of aging but they can also be indicators of something deeper, like early dementia or depression. Don't be afraid to trust your instincts. You know your loved one.

If you're beginning to notice changes, this is a good time to start having gentle conversations. Not everything needs to be solved overnight. In fact, it's best if it's not. Begin by checking in more often. Offer to help with small things like managing the mail or cooking a meal together.

It may also be a good time to schedule a medical appointment, not necessarily to make a diagnosis, but to begin documenting any cognitive, emotional, or physical changes. Early detection can lead to better management, more options, and peace of mind.

When your loved one forgets something important like a birthday, a familiar name, or a recent event, it can be tempting to ask, "Don't you remember?" But this question, though well-intentioned, can unintentionally cause shame or frustration. For someone with memory loss, it may highlight what they can no longer access, leaving them feeling confused or "less than."

Instead, gently supply the memory without putting pressure on them:
- Instead of: "Don't you remember Sarah came yesterday?"
  Try: "Sarah came by yesterday. She brought your favorite muffins. You smiled the whole time."
- Instead of: "We already talked about this, remember?"
  Try: "Let me share it with you again. It's no problem."

These small shifts in language can protect their dignity and maintain the warmth in your relationship. Remember, your tone and patience speak louder than your words.

Watching a parent or loved one change can bring up deep feelings like grief, fear, confusion, even guilt. These emotions are real and valid. You are witnessing someone you love navigate a shift that neither of you expected, and that's a powerful experience. Give yourself grace as you adjust, and allow room for your own care in the process.

I once had a client who was one of the sweetest, most proper ladies I've ever cared for. She had the elegance of a time gone by. She was graceful, composed, and incredibly thoughtful. She came from the generation that didn't waste anything and believed in the power of routine. Her favorite midnight ritual was sneaking into the kitchen for a bowl of Raisin Bran, which she swore by for "keeping things regular."

Now, I already knew Raisin Bran had its digestive benefits. But this particular morning, I learned just how effective it could be.

She was mobile and independent enough to roam safely at night, so it wasn't unusual for her to quietly enjoy her cereal and go back to bed. But when I awakened that morning, I was hit with… let's just say… the aftermath. It looked like a battlefield of bran and dignity, and I stood frozen at the door, trying to process the sheer scope of what had occurred. Her bed was empty. The floor… not so much. It seemed she had relocated herself to another bedroom. Smart move. When I found her, she was looking as serene as an early spring morning.

I asked gently, "Mrs. E, do you know what happened last night?"

She looked me dead in the eyes, sweet as pie, and said with all the innocence in the world, "Oh no, honey. I don't know who did that but it certainly wasn't me."

At that moment, all I could do was laugh and grab the gloves.

These are the moments that catch you off guard. The ones that are messy and real and sometimes downright hilarious. But they're also reminders that this journey may be about loss but it's also about love, humanity, and yes, even humor. It's okay to laugh. It's okay to cry. And it's always okay to extend grace to both your loved one and yourself.

One practical way to help both your loved one and their medical providers is to keep a small journal of your observations. Note things such as:

- Changes in mood or behavior
- Missed appointments or tasks
- Changes in hygiene, grooming, or appetite

- Repeated stories or confusion with dates and time

This is not meant to be clinical; it's a loving tool to help you keep track of patterns. It may also help you communicate more clearly with doctors or other caregivers as time goes on.

Chapter 3

HELPING THEM FEEL SAFE

When someone begins to struggle with memory, daily tasks, or even confusion about time or place, their world can start to feel unpredictable. Things that once came easily now require effort. This change can feel frightening and isolating for your loved one, even if they don't or can't say it aloud.

As a caregiver or family member, one of the most powerful gifts you can offer is a sense of safety. Not just physical safety but emotional, mental, and spiritual peace.

Routines give structure to the day and structure brings comfort. Whether your loved one is living independently, with family, or in a care setting, having familiar touchstones throughout the day helps reduce anxiety and confusion.

Try to keep mealtimes, medication times, walks, or favorite shows consistent. Even something as simple as offering coffee in the same mug or playing soft music during breakfast can create an anchor of normalcy.

Routines don't need to be rigid. Flexibility is key. The goal is rhythm, not strict scheduling.

As memory fades, the world around your loved one can begin to feel unfamiliar, even their own home or family members. It's common for them to ask the same questions repeatedly or become agitated when they don't recognize someone or something.

Here's where your response becomes vital. Your voice, your words, and your expressions will become their safety net. Therefore, be mindful in these ways:

- Speak slowly, clearly, and warmly.
- Don't argue or correct in a way that makes them feel "wrong."
- Validate their feelings, even if they're based on a misremembered event.

Instead of: "No, that didn't happen."

Try: "I can see that upset you. I'm here now, and you're safe."

These small changes can defuse stress and bring comfort in moments of confusion.

If you're having a hard time getting cooperation, whether it's with bathing, eating, or another activity, and the mood or temperature starts to escalate, it's okay to take a step back. Don't try to force things in a moment of high emotion.

Backing away for a little while gives both of you a chance to reset. Often, just stepping out of the room or shifting focus can help calm the atmosphere. After some time, you can try again with a softer, more patient tone or approach the situation differently.

Redirection is another powerful tool. If your loved one becomes fixated or agitated, gently redirect their attention to something comforting or familiar like a photo album, a snack, a walk, or soft music. Sometimes it's not about fixing the problem; it's about gently guiding attention toward something more peaceful.

More than ever, your loved one needs someone in their corner. As their memory or ability to communicate changes, they may become vulnerable to being overlooked, misunderstood, or even taken advantage of. Unfortunately, the elderly are often targets for neglect, fraud, or subpar care, and many no longer have the tools to speak up for themselves.

That's why being an advocate is one of your most important roles.
- Speak up at doctor's appointments if something doesn't seem right.
- Ask questions about medications or treatments.
- Review insurance, billing, and care plans carefully.
- Be present and vocal when dealing with care facilities, agencies, or home aides.

Your attention to detail and your willingness to stand up for them could make all the difference in their well-being and dignity.

Being an advocate also means knowing their preferences and honoring their voice even if they can't always express it clearly. Watch their body language. Listen with your heart. You may be the only one who truly understands how they feel, what they like, and what brings them comfort. For many older adults, especially those with dementia or Alzheimer's, gentle touch can be deeply calming. A warm hand on theirs, a hug, or a soft pat on the back may say more than any words. You can also support emotional safety by designing a calming environment:
- Lighting: Keep rooms well-lit but not harsh.
- Noise: Reduce background noise and overstimulation.
- Smells: Use soft, familiar scents like lavender, lemon, or cinnamon (essential oils can help).
- Photos: Display family photos or items from their past to anchor them to their story.

Processing time slows down with age or cognitive changes. If you ask a question or give instructions, allow time for them to respond. Don't rush them. The pause might feel long to you, but they may still be forming their answer.

Also, simplify choices. Instead of asking, "What do you want to wear today?", try: "Would you like the blue sweater or the gray one?" Small moments like this build confidence and preserve dignity.

I once cared for a client who absolutely hated taking showers. That's not uncommon in the world of Alzheimer's. Many feel vulnerable, confused, or simply afraid of the process. When I began caring for her, she was living in a facility and, heartbreakingly, hadn't had a real shower in nearly two months. But, I could tell there was more to her. She had once loved fashion. But now her coordination and memory had faded. I decided to make bathing less about the task and more about her. We started with the closet. Together, we picked out beautiful outfits, things that lit up her eyes and made her sit a little taller. Then we'd sit at her vanity, and I'd talk to her about doing her hair, a bit of makeup, and how lovely she would look once she felt fresh and clean. I made it an experience, not a chore. There was always dignity in the details: mats on the shower floor, warm towels waiting, and each step explained before it happened. I showed her I was there. Present. Patient. Safe.

And something amazing happened. The resistance faded. The fear softened. Soon, showers became smooth, and I honestly think she began to look forward to them. It wasn't just about cleanliness. She was remembering herself. Her style. Her beauty. Her worth.

Week by week, I watched her transform physically and emotionally. The woman who once seemed so unkempt began to glow. She bloomed. And these are the moments that remind me why I do this work. When we care with dignity, we bring people back to life in the most sacred ways.

Creating space for your loved one to feel safe also helps them to breathe, rest, trust and be themselves. Even in moments of confusion or frustration, your presence, patience, and compassion are powerful medicine. You may not get it all right but as you show up day after day, your steady heart becomes the light that guides them safely through the fog.

Chapter 4

THE POWER OF MUSIC & NATURE IN HEALING

Healing doesn't always begin with a pill or a procedure. Sometimes, it begins with a soft melody, a gentle breeze, the scent of lavender drifting through a room, or even the quiet act of brushing someone's hair. For our aging loved ones, especially those battling memory loss, Alzheimer's, or dementia, these moments of connection to the natural world and to the heart can bring more peace than words ever could. We often underestimate the power of what seems simple. But in caregiving, simplicity can be profound.

I once had a client who had been a real estate mogul, but her current state seemed far removed from that chapter of her life. Such a powerful woman was now afraid from moment to moment. This was one of the times I was allowed to introduce scented oils like lavender and peppermint. These calming aromas seemed to reach parts of her soul that words couldn't. There was a noticeable difference in her mood and her cooperation. It reminded me that healing doesn't always require speaking. Sometimes, it begins with the air we breathe and the love we bring into a room.

I had another client who I introduced to music, and those sessions became the highlight of her day. She had a disease similar to Parkinson's, and I could tell that music allowed her to escape from the focus on her pain. Music has a way of making us feel alive again. It gave her purpose, joy, and a space to simply be herself.

There is something extraordinary about music. It bypasses damaged parts of the brain and goes straight to the heart. In dementia and Alzheimer's care, music often evokes memories long forgotten. A familiar song from childhood, a hymn they sang in church, or a tune they danced to in their youth can unlock smiles, laughter, and tears.

- Reduce agitation and anxiety
- Improve mood and emotional well-being
- Encourage movement and participation
- Create moments of shared joy and recognition

You don't need a trained therapist to begin using music in your caregiving routine. Just observe what resonates. Use playlists from the era your loved one grew up in. Keep the volume soft and allow moments of silence for rest and reflection. Sing with them if they enjoy it. Music is even more powerful when it's shared.

Nature therapy, or ecotherapy, is a deeply restorative tool. Being outdoors, even for a few minutes a day, can significantly improve mental and emotional health. For those with limited mobility, even sitting near a window that overlooks trees, flowers, or birds can shift their entire mood.

- Lower blood pressure and stress hormones
- Improve mood and reduce depression
- Spark joy and engagement
- Provide natural light to help regulate sleep patterns
- A short walk in the garden
- Sitting on the porch with a cup of tea
- Listening to birdsong under a shaded tree
- Tending to plants or watering flowers

Incorporating herbs, supplements, and essential oils can be another layer of support. Many elderly individuals respond positively to these gentle therapies, especially when they are tailored to their needs.
- Lavender & Chamomile Oil – Promotes calm and sleep
- Peppermint Oil – Uplifting and may aid alertness
- Rosemary & Lemon – Traditionally associated with memory support
- Marshmallow Root, Uva Ursi, and Cranberry – Support urinary tract health

Always consult a healthcare professional before adding herbs or oils, especially when your loved one is on medications. But don't dismiss the power of a lavender-scented room at bedtime or a warm peppermint oil rub on sore joints.

Touch is one of the most powerful forms of connection. Gentle acts like brushing your loved one's hair, styling it, or giving them a facial or manicure are more than just grooming, they're ways to preserve dignity and create closeness.

A spa day doesn't have to be expensive or elaborate. It can be as simple as:
- A warm hair wash followed by gentle brushing and styling
- Soaking hands in warm water with essential oils and massaging with lotion
- Trimming and painting nails with their favorite color
- Looking through old family photos together and talking about cherished memories

Every person is different. What calms one may irritate another. What brings joy to one may bring confusion to someone else. That's why personalized care is so important. Get to know what your loved one enjoys. Study them. Notice the small things that make them feel at home in their own body and mind.

Caregiving is not a checklist. It's a relationship. The small gestures, like the flowers from outside placed on their nightstand, the old family recipe you cook together, the fresh air shared during a quiet moment on a bench, are the memories that linger and make a difference.

Music, nature, herbs, and heartfelt care are not mere luxuries. They are necessities. Especially for those losing their grip on memory or identity. These healing tools remind them, and us, that they are still connected to something beautiful. And sometimes, when words fail, it's the scent of rosemary, the sound of birdsong, or the rhythm of a favorite hymn that speaks straight to the soul.

Chapter 5

CHOOSING THE RIGHT CAREGIVER OR COMPANION

I, as a caregiver, have been on both sides of the selection process. I've managed memory care facilities and supported families looking for someone they could trust with their most precious person. Let me tell you, it's not easy. Attempting to find a caring, motivated caregiver can be a daunting task. The job has to come from the heart or it just doesn't work.

As an empathic soul myself, I can spot another empath almost immediately. But even then, sometimes you have to go through a dozen applicants to find one who truly possesses all the qualities needed—not just skill, but soul. Take your time. This is someone who will not only be a helper but a witness to some of the most vulnerable and sacred moments in your loved one's life.

As a caregiver, be the person the family has been waiting for. Let your presence be a comfort, your heart be steady, and your spirit be humble. This kind of approach creates long-lasting relationships that bless both the client and the caregiver. Caregivers, set yourself apart. Learn what makes a great caregiver even if it doesn't come naturally at first. With intention and heart, it can be learned.

Choosing a caregiver is one of the most important decisions you will make in your loved one's care journey. This person won't just assist with tasks, they will share quiet moments, comfort during vulnerability, and often become part of the family. That's why it's so important to approach this step with both your head and your heart.

A good caregiver brings more than skills. They also bring presence, patience, and compassion. They're able to respond to needs, adjust to moods, and offer stability and reassurance. Look for someone who is not only trained or certified (if needed) but also genuinely interested in caring for others. You want someone who sees your loved one as a person, not a job.

- Patience, especially in moments of repetition or confusion
- Consistency and reliability
- Good communication with both the client and family
- Flexibility, especially with changing routines
- A warm, respectful tone that preserves dignity

Don't be afraid to interview multiple caregivers. Ask questions about their experience, especially with memory loss or dementia, if applicable. Observe how they interact with your loved one. Do they speak directly to them? Do they smile or listen with empathy?

Start with a trial period when possible. The best matches often reveal themselves through simple moments such as how they handle a question, help with a meal, or manage a rough day.

It's important to remember that not every caregiver is right for every client. Even the most skilled caregiver may not be the right fit for your loved one. That doesn't mean they're not good at what they do. It just may be a mismatch in personality, communication style, or preferences.

Some clients prefer male caregivers; others feel safer with females. Some love chatty, upbeat personalities, while others prefer a calm, quiet presence. That's okay. These dynamics matter.

It goes both ways. The caregiver also needs to feel comfortable and supported by the family. Kindness, mutual respect, and communication are key. A successful caregiving relationship happens when both parties feel safe, appreciated, and happy in the space they share.

When in doubt, ask:
- Does my loved one seem more calm or more anxious with this person?
- Is the caregiver able to meet needs without being overwhelmed?
- Is the communication open and respectful?

A caregiver who is respected and valued will naturally give better care.

Pay attention to how your loved one responds over time. Also, stay in conversation with the caregiver. Do they feel equipped? Supported? Sometimes a caregiver may also sense that the relationship isn't a good match and that's worth listening to.

You want your loved one to thrive, and you want the caregiver to thrive too. A relationship built on balance, mutual respect, and good communication is more likely to last and to enrich everyone involved.

Chapter 6

WHEN YOUR LOVED ONE MOVES INTO ASSISTED LIVING

Moving a loved one into assisted living is never a light decision. It often comes after months, sometimes years, of weighing options, watching changes, and realizing that more help is needed than you or others can safely provide at home. Even when you know it's the right move, it can stir up emotions like guilt, sadness, and uncertainty.

But assisted living doesn't mean the end of connection or care. In many cases, it becomes the beginning of a new chapter where your loved one receives the support they need, and you regain the emotional space to be present as family, not just as a caregiver.

WEIGHING ALL YOUR OPTIONS

Assisted living isn't a one-size-fits-all solution. Every family is different and so is every elder's personality and comfort level. Before making a final decision, consider all possible environments that may provide the right balance of care, comfort, and connection.

One alternative is a residential care home, often nestled in quiet neighborhoods. These smaller settings provide an intimate environment that feels more like being in a private home. The limited number of residents fosters deeper relationships, not just with caregivers, but also with fellow residents. In many of these homes, the staff becomes like family, offering consistent and attentive care in a setting that feels cozy, personal, and safe.

Another option is in-home care, which allows your loved one to remain in their familiar environment, surrounded by their own belongings, routines, and memories. With the help of skilled caregivers brought into the home, this setup can offer a high level of comfort and emotional stability, particularly if your loved one is resistant to leaving home. If your family's budget allows, this route can offer highly personalized care while preserving independence.

Tip: Consider reaching out to placement agencies such as A Place for Mom, which can help identify residential care homes or other local care options based on your loved one's needs and personality.

Ultimately, the best choice is the one that honors your loved one's preferences while meeting their evolving care needs. Safety, comfort, and dignity should guide the decision.

EASING THE TRANSITION

The first few weeks are often the hardest for both the resident and their family. Your loved one may express sadness, fear, or even resentment. These feelings are normal. It's a big adjustment, especially for those used to their own routines and surroundings.

Here's how you can ease the transition:
- Familiar items: Bring in their favorite chair, blankets, framed photos, or keepsakes to make the room feel like home.
- Routine visits: Visit consistently, especially at the beginning. Help establish a sense of familiarity in the new environment.

- Meet the staff: Introduce yourself to caregivers, nurses, and aides. Let them know personal preferences, routines, and personality traits of your loved one.
- Stay positive: Your attitude sets the tone. Speak with warmth and encouragement, even if it's difficult at first.

THE IMPORTANCE OF COMMUNICATION

Keep communication open between you, the facility, and your loved one. Ask questions. Request updates. Attend family meetings or care plan reviews. Don't hesitate to advocate if something seems off or if your loved one is having a hard time adjusting.

Also, encourage your loved one to express their feelings. Even if they can't articulate everything clearly, your attention and empathy will help them feel less alone.

WHAT ACTIVITIES ARE OFFERED?

Most assisted living communities offer daily and weekly activities designed to keep residents socially engaged, physically active, and mentally stimulated.

Common activities include:
- Arts and crafts
- Music and singalongs
- Chair yoga or gentle exercise classes
- Gardening
- Card games and puzzles
- Devotional or religious services
- Outings to parks, events, or restaurants

Ask for the activity calendar and see what your loved one might enjoy. Encourage participation but don't push too hard. There are some days when they may prefer quiet time, and that's okay too.

CONTINUE YOUR BOND IN NEW WAYS

Even though you're no longer providing direct daily care, your role is still incredibly meaningful. You are still their safe space, their advocate, their familiar voice.

Here are ways to stay connected:
- Bring their favorite snacks or homemade meals.
- Sit with them during meals or activities.
- Take them for walks or spend time in the garden.
- Bring photo albums or create new ones together.
- Celebrate small holidays and birthdays with simple decorations or treats.
- Even a short visit can brighten their entire day.

BE PATIENT WITH YOURSELF, TOO

Families often carry guilt when they place a loved one into assisted living even if it's the safest and most logical step. It's okay to grieve what once was. But remind yourself that you are still caring; you're just doing it differently now.

This decision can allow both of you to breathe again. It offers your loved one consistency and safety, and it offers you the chance to restore your own health and well-being, which is just as important.

CLOSING THOUGHT

Moving into assisted living, or any form of long-term care, is a major transition. But it doesn't have to be the end of joy, connection, or dignity. With continued love, thoughtful involvement, and open communication, this new chapter can still be filled with meaning, peace, and precious moments together.

Chapter 7

WHEN A CAREGIVER BECOMES FAMILY

At some point during the caregiving journey, a shift often happens that is felt more than it is seen. A hired caregiver is no longer just someone who helps with meals or medications. They become a trusted companion, a source of comfort, a steady presence in times of change. In many families, that caregiver becomes part of the family.

This bond is not built overnight. It grows from shared routines, long conversations, and quiet moments of understanding. And when it happens, it's a blessing, not just for your loved one, but for the entire family.

Good caregivers don't simply clock in and out. They give of themselves in ways that often go unseen. They soothe fears that arise in the middle of the night. They stay calm when tempers flare or confusion sets in. They listen to the same stories again and again and still smile. They celebrate small victories (a full meal eaten, a restful nap, a kind word spoken).

What many people forget is that caregivers also carry emotional weight along with physical duties. They form bonds, feel losses, and pour from their own cup daily. And often, they are doing this while raising their own children, supporting their families, or managing personal challenges.

This is why recognizing the caregiver's humanity is so essential. They are both helpers and healers. They bring their full hearts into the work. If your caregiver has become part of your loved one's life, it's important to nurture that bond with mutual respect. Appreciation doesn't always need to be extravagant. It can be:
- A heartfelt thank-you note or small gift
- Including them in celebrations or holiday meals (if they're open to it)
- Checking in on how they're doing, not just what they're doing
- Respecting their off-time and personal boundaries
- A caregiver who feels valued is more likely to stay and more likely to pour love into every action. The family should remember that a good caregiver needs care too. They usually give, give, and give and give some more. But their cup needs refilling. Caregivers are often:
- Underpaid for the emotional and physical labor they provide
- Overworked due to long hours and staff shortages
- Emotionally drained from witnessing decline or managing tough behaviors

When you have a good caregiver, honor that. Pay fairly when possible. Advocate for proper breaks. Give grace during hard days. Because this person is helping you carry one of the most sacred responsibilities, the loving and caring for someone you love. Great caregiving involves a true partnership between the caregiver and the family. Communication, trust, and shared goals create the foundation.

Check in regularly:
- "Is there anything we can do to make your job easier?"
- "How is Mom doing from your perspective?"
- "Are there any supplies or tools you need?"

- These simple questions go a long way in building respect and reducing burnout. When everyone feels seen, safe, and appreciated, caregiving transforms from a task into a deeply fulfilling relationship.

When a caregiver becomes family, something beautiful happens. The work becomes care for sure but beyond that, it becomes connection. And just like your loved one deserves to be honored in their later years, so does the one who walks beside them.

Take care of your caregiver. Cherish their presence. Celebrate the love they bring into your home. Because sometimes, the greatest gift you can give your loved one… is the person who helps them feel safe, respected, and loved every single day.

Chapter 8

SELECTING AN ASSISTED LIVING COMMUNITY OR RESIDENTIAL CARE HOME

Choosing where your loved one will live during their later years is one of the most significant decisions a family can make. Safety or logistics are important but so is the quality of life, dignity, and peace of mind for everyone involved. Whether you're searching for a traditional assisted living community or a smaller residential care home, the goal is always the same: finding the right fit for your loved one's needs, personality, and preferences.

Before touring locations or making calls, take a moment to assess what your loved one truly needs. Likewise, think about your own needs as a family caregiver. How close do you want to be to their new residence? Are you looking for a place where you can visit often? Will you need flexibility with visiting hours or involvement in care planning? Being clear on needs from the beginning will help you avoid feeling overwhelmed by too many options. Traditional Assisted Living Communities often offer more amenities and structured activities. These facilities may include:

- On-site dining services
- Group activities and outings

- Fitness classes or wellness programs
- Medical staff on-call or nearby
- Residential Care Homes, also known as board and care homes, offer a more intimate setting, often with as few as three or four residents in a house nestled within a residential neighborhood. These homes may feel more personal and home-like.

Benefits include:
- Lower staff-to-resident ratios
- Familiar, cozy environment
- More personalized attention
- Family-like atmosphere

For many families, a smaller home can feel like an extension of their own household. The caregivers become like extended family members, and the atmosphere is warm and less institutional. Some residents thrive in this close-knit setting.

There is also the option of in-home care if your loved one prefers to stay in their current home. While this may not be sustainable long-term for every family, it is a viable option, especially when paired with home health services or live-in care. If financially feasible, this allows your loved one to remain in familiar surroundings and avoid a major transition.

A placement agency like A Place For Mom can be a helpful resource in finding smaller residential homes or evaluating different care settings that fit your needs. Once you have a list of places to consider, visit each one and bring a checklist. Trust your gut, but also take notes.

- Is the staff warm, respectful, and attentive?
- Do the residents appear content and engaged?
- Are there smells of food or unpleasant odors?
- Is the facility clean, safe, and well-maintained?
- Are there outdoor areas for walking or sitting?
- What kinds of activities are scheduled weekly?

- How do they handle medical emergencies?

Ask to see the daily activity calendar and meal menu. Look at common spaces and private rooms. Observe interactions between staff and residents.

If possible, visit more than once and drop in unexpectedly during different times of day. You'll get a more accurate picture of what life is really like there.

A beautiful building means nothing if your loved one feels isolated or uncomfortable. Think about:
- Does the environment reflect your loved one's personality?
- Will they feel out of place, or at ease?
- Would they want to connect with the other residents?
- Are there cultural or faith-based components that matter to your family?

You want more than a safe place. You want a fitting place. Whenever possible, involve your loved one in the process, even if only in small ways. Give them choices. Let them tour with you. Ask what feels comfortable to them. Even if they can't articulate exactly what they want, their body language and reactions will tell you a lot.

Empowering them with a voice in this transition helps preserve their dignity and reduces anxiety about the unknown. The right care setting is one where your loved one can feel safe, seen, and supported and where you, as a family member, feel peace. Don't rush the process. Ask questions, follow your instincts, and remember: You're not only finding a place; you're choosing a home.

Chapter 9

THE POWER OF HOLISTIC HEALING – HERBS, OILS, SUPPLEMENTS & MORE

Caring for a loved one involves managing symptoms for sure. But it's crucial to understand that it's also about nurturing the whole person: mind, body, and spirit. While medications have their place, many caregivers discover that holistic approaches can provide gentle, powerful support for aging individuals, especially those facing chronic conditions, memory loss, or emotional distress.

These methods are not meant to replace traditional medicine but to complement it, adding warmth, comfort, and balance to daily care. Long before pharmaceutical companies, people turned to herbs to ease pain, promote rest, and support healing. Our elderly loved ones may benefit from some of these same natural remedies when used responsibly.

Some herbs and supplements that support aging and cognitive wellness:
- Ginkgo Biloba – May improve circulation and support memory function.
- Turmeric/Curcumin – An anti-inflammatory that may help with joint pain and brain health.

- Ashwagandha – An adaptogen that can help reduce stress and support the nervous system.
- Fish Oil (Omega-3s) – Known for supporting brain and heart health.
- Vitamin D and B12 – Often deficient in older adults and important for mood and memory.
- Marshmallow Root, Uva Ursi, and Cranberry – Especially helpful for urinary tract health, which is critical as UTIs in seniors can lead to confusion, memory changes, and agitation.

Always consult a healthcare provider before adding herbs or supplements, especially if your loved one takes medications. Some herbs can interact with prescriptions or affect blood pressure, liver function, or blood sugar levels.

The scent of lavender in a quiet room. A warm cloth infused with peppermint oil placed on the forehead. These aren't luxuries. They are acts of love that soothe the senses and support emotional well-being.

Some favorite essential oils in eldercare:
- Lavender – Calms anxiety, supports sleep, reduces agitation.
- Peppermint – Uplifts mood, relieves headaches, supports digestion.
- Rosemary – Often used in memory care for alertness and focus.
- Lemon – Refreshing and cleansing; may support mental clarity.
- Frankincense – Promotes deep breathing, spiritual calm, and focus.

Ways to use essential oils:
- Diffuse in the room for 20–30 minutes at a time.
- Mix a few drops with carrier oil (like coconut or almond oil) for massage.
- Add to warm bath water for relaxation (only if safe for your loved one).
- Apply a drop to a handkerchief for them to hold or sniff when agitated.

Food and drink are foundational to holistic care. A balanced diet rich in whole foods, vegetables, fruits, fiber, and good fats, supports all systems of the body, especially the brain.

- Natural teas can be used to calm and comfort.
- Chamomile – Promotes sleep and digestion.
- Lemon Balm – Supports mood and reduces stress.
- Ginger – Soothes the stomach and supports circulation.
- Hibiscus – May lower blood pressure and offer a gentle lift.

These teas also create rituals. A warm cup before bed. A morning moment on the porch. These are healing, too.

Holistic caregiving doesn't mean you have to do everything all at once. It's about bringing awareness to how every sense, sight, smell, sound, touch, and taste can be part of care.

Ask yourself:

- How does their space smell? Is it inviting and clean?
- Are there calming sounds like music, water, or birds?
- Are their meals colorful, fresh, and lovingly prepared?
- Is their room filled with natural light or comforting lamps?
- Do they feel seen, heard, and held?

Even if memory fades, the body remembers love.

Herbs, oils, supplements, music, and nature… these tools are more than "extras." They are deeply rooted in humanity's oldest healing practices. And in the hands of a loving caregiver, they can provide comfort, reduce distress, and create beautiful moments of peace and joy.

In holistic care, we see the person as well as the diagnosis. We treat the whole being, not merely the symptoms. Because healing isn't always about fixing; it's about honoring.

Chapter 10

TIPS FOR SELECTING A CAREGIVER

Finding the right caregiver is one of the most important steps you'll take on this caregiving journey. The right person won't only help with tasks; they'll become a companion, a trusted presence, and often, an extension of the family. This chapter is about hiring someone who will treat your loved one with dignity, patience, and heart.

Before beginning the search, take time to list your family's specific needs. This will guide your conversations and interviews later.

Ask yourself:
- What tasks will the caregiver need to perform? (e.g., bathing, dressing, meal prep, medication reminders)
- Will the caregiver need a driver's license or transportation?
- Will this be full-time, part-time, live-in, or a few hours a week?
- Does your loved one require someone with experience in dementia or mobility care?

Being specific helps you avoid misunderstandings and ensures everyone is on the same page from the beginning.

There are a few routes you can take:

- Home Care Agencies: They screen, train, and manage caregivers, but often at a higher cost.
- Independent Caregivers: You can hire privately through recommendations, local caregiver networks, or platforms like Care.com.
- Referrals: Word of mouth can be invaluable. Ask friends, neighbors, church members, or medical providers if they know someone trustworthy.

If hiring independently, be sure to conduct background checks, ask for references, and discuss expectations in writing.

Meeting a caregiver for the first time is an opportunity to go beyond their resume. What do you sense about their spirit. Look for warmth, patience, and a willingness to learn about your loved one as a person.

Questions to ask:
- What experience do you have with elderly or memory-impaired individuals?
- How do you handle someone who's having a difficult or agitated day?
- What is your philosophy of caregiving?
- Can you provide personal references?
- Are you open to being trained in how our family handles specific routines or preferences?

Also, observe how they interact with your loved one. Does your loved one feel comfortable? Are they respectful, gentle, and attentive?

It's important to understand that just because a caregiver is skilled doesn't mean they'll be the right match for your family and that's okay.

Sometimes a caregiver might be a perfect fit for one individual, and not for another. That doesn't make them a bad caregiver. It may simply mean their personality or style doesn't align with your loved one's needs or history. Some clients prefer male caregivers, others prefer females. Cultural differences, communication styles, or even energy levels can all play a role.

A good match means:
- Your loved one feels safe and respected
- The caregiver feels appreciated and heard
- The overall home atmosphere is peaceful

Always consider both sides. You want a happy loved one and a happy caregiver working together in a safe, respectful space. That's how lasting relationships are built.

Even if everything looks great on paper, consider starting with a short trial period, maybe a week or two, to see how things go. This allows both your loved one and the caregiver to ease into the relationship without pressure.

During this time, check in often. Be honest about what's working and what's not, and invite the caregiver to do the same. Open communication from the beginning helps build trust and resolve concerns early.

Watch for these qualities:
- Reliability: They show up on time and follow through.
- Compassion: They genuinely care, not just complete tasks.
- Flexibility: They can adapt to your loved one's changing needs or moods.
- Respect: They honor your loved one's dignity, space, and history.
- Communication: They update you regularly and are easy to talk to.

Being a caregiver is a hard and often underappreciated job. Good caregivers pour themselves out daily, physically, emotionally, spiritually. When you find a good one, take care of them, too.
- Say thank you often.
- Check in and ask how they are doing.
- Offer time off when possible.
- Pay fairly and on time.
- Celebrate milestones and build a respectful relationship.

When caregivers feel supported, they give even more from the heart.

Choosing the right caregiver is a partnership, one rooted in trust, compassion, and respect. Don't rush the process. The right match can make all the difference in your loved one's well-being and your peace of mind.

And when you find that special person, the one who shows up, stays present, and treats your loved one like their own, hold onto them. They are rare, and they are a blessing.

Chapter 11

A CAREGIVER'S HEART – A GENTLE REMINDER TO FAMILIES

Behind every clean shirt, every hot meal, every midnight reassurance, and every soft-spoken redirection… is a caregiver with a full heart and often, an empty tank. Caregiving is more than a job. It truly is a mission deeply grounded in love. And when a caregiver becomes part of your loved one's world, they often give more than time. They give themselves.

This chapter is a gentle but important reminder: caregivers need care too.

When you find someone who truly connects with your loved one, who sees them as a whole person, not just a task list, you've found more than a worker. You've found a partner. Many families are surprised at how deeply a bond can form. That caregiver may be the one your loved one calls for in moments of confusion or joy. They may know the right song to sing when your loved one is anxious, or how to soothe them with a joke and a warm blanket.

They are not 'just an aide.' They are often the reason your loved one smiles that day.

That bond deserves to be seen and honored.

Good caregivers pour from their emotional cup every single day. They absorb the stress of someone else's pain, behaviors, and decline while keeping themselves steady. They may go home to their own families, their own struggles, and still show up for yours with kindness and grace.

But too often, caregivers are undervalued or overlooked. They are expected to handle everything with endless patience, even when they are exhausted. They're asked to go above and beyond without thanks or fair compensation.

So here's what you can do:
- Say thank you often – Small words, big impact. A sincere note, text, or spoken thank you can lift someone's spirit more than you realize.
- Respect their time – Avoid last-minute changes or assumptions. Treat their schedule with the same respect as any professional.
- Give breaks – Everyone needs time to reset. If your caregiver is live-in or works long hours, build in time off or rest days.
- Pay fairly – If you've found someone wonderful, compensate them accordingly. They're not just filling a position; they're sustaining your family's peace.
- Celebrate them – Acknowledge birthdays, holidays, or work anniversaries. Make them feel seen.

Caregiving is emotional labor. Whether it's tears over a lost memory or laughter during a shared story, it all takes energy. And just like any of us, caregivers need to be refilled in order to continue giving.

Encourage your caregiver to take care of themselves:
- Ask them how they are doing.
- Support their personal and professional goals.
- Offer moments of quiet when possible.
- Speak kindly. Be patient with their humanness.

Remember: A well-supported caregiver is a better caregiver.

So much of caregiving goes unseen:
- The way they talk gently even when no one responds.
- The countless diapers changed or meals reheated.
- The moments spent waiting patiently for a confused mind to find its words.
- The times they cried in silence after witnessing someone's decline.

When you acknowledge the invisible, you validate their effort. And that validation is priceless.

To all the families reading this: when you find someone who loves your loved one like you do, hold onto them. Take care of them. Protect them.

Because caregivers are underpaid and often underappreciated, but they are delivering one of the most sacred services in the world: human dignity, comfort, and presence.

And that is something worth cherishing.

Chapter 12

ALZHEIMER'S AND DEMENTIA – HOME HEALTH CARE & HOPE

When a loved one is diagnosed with Alzheimer's or dementia, the world can suddenly feel unfamiliar for them and for you. Memory lapses, confusion, mood swings, and the gradual loss of independence can be overwhelming to witness. But you're not alone, and neither is your loved one. There are tools, people, and services that can help shoulder the weight and home health care is one of them.

Alzheimer's and other forms of dementia affect the brain in complex ways, gradually changing how a person thinks, communicates, remembers, and behaves. These changes aren't linear, and each person's journey is different. Some days may feel normal, while others may feel like the person you love is slipping away.

What remains constant, though, is your love and your ability to advocate for them, guide them gently, and support them through the shifting tides.

Common challenges include:
- Repeating questions or stories

- Disorientation about time, place, or people
- Difficulty performing familiar tasks

Home health care can offer tremendous relief and guidance. A skilled and compassionate caregiver can support both physical and emotional needs, allowing your loved one to age in place safely, with dignity. From medication management and hygiene assistance to companionship and memory support, home care professionals can help lighten your daily load.

When looking for home health services, consider agencies with experience in dementia care. Ask about caregiver training, consistency, and how they handle changes in behavior or mood.

Helpful directories such as Caring.com can help you locate reputable agencies in your area, read reviews, and compare services.

Chapter 13

WHEN THE SUN GOES DOWN – MEETING THE SOUL AT DUSK

As the light fades and shadows begin to stretch across the room, something quiet and unsettling often stirs in our loved ones. What should feel like a peaceful close to the day may instead bring confusion, fear, or even resistance.

This is sundowning.

And for caregivers, it is one of the most emotionally delicate hours of the day.

Sundowning is a symptom of dementia or Alzheimer's where restlessness, agitation, or disorientation increases in the late afternoon or early evening. It can look different from one person to the next. Some may pace or cry. Others may grow suspicious or even aggressive. They might say, *"I want to go home,"* even when they're sitting in their own living room.

This isn't your loved one turning against you. It's their mind struggling to interpret a world that no longer feels familiar.

Sundowning is something I've witnessed more times than I can count, and yet it never gets easier. Each person is different, but the behaviors are so often the same. A shift in the air, a look of fear in the eyes, the anxious movement of hands searching for keys or a coat. The sun begins to set, and suddenly the person you've known so well is ready to leave, determined to go "home." But home isn't always where they live now. Sometimes it's a memory, a feeling, or a time long passed.

One of the most heart-wrenching experiences I had with sundowning was with someone very close to me—a family member who was strong, poised, and fiercely independent her whole life. She was the type of woman who commanded respect when she walked into a room. Her identity was deeply tied to her work and her career had been her purpose, her pride, her sanctuary.

As her mind began to slip, slowly at first, we tried to rationalize it. We chalked up the little things to aging, stress, or just "having a lot on her mind." But the signs were there. We just didn't want to see them.

Then it started happening. Just as the day began to fade into night, she would grab her purse, find her keys, and drive downtown to the office she had retired from years ago. To her, that was home. That job, that space, those memories were a part of who she was. And when the world around her no longer made sense, that's where her heart told her to go.

For a while, she would circle around, confused but somehow always making it back. Until one night, she didn't. The fear that gripped our hearts that night was unforgettable. She was found safely, thank God, but things changed after that. The car keys had to be taken away, and we had to start thinking about how to keep her safe in ways that broke our hearts. Her independence, the very thing she had always valued, was slowly being replaced by confusion, anxiety, and fear.

She also began hiding her jewelry, family heirlooms, anything she deemed important. These items became symbols of security in a world that was becoming unfamiliar. And when she couldn't find them later, the panic would return.

Sundowning is more than confusion in the evening hours. There is a loss of time, of clarity, of control. And you're watching someone you love drift between moments of lucidity and fear. And as a caregiver, it tests your patience, your strength, and your heart in the most sacred of ways.

But I also learned that in those moments, love matters most. A gentle voice, a reassuring hand, soft lighting, familiar music, and simply being present can sometimes anchor them, even if just for a moment. Sundowning taught me to listen with my eyes and my heart, not just my ears. It taught me to meet them where they are, not where I wish they still were.

This story, like so many others, lives in my heart as a reminder that caregiving involves preserving dignity, honoring stories, and loving someone through the fog.

Our internal body clock, our circadian rhythm, relies on light, routine, and predictability. Dementia disrupts that rhythm. As daylight wanes and the environment shifts, confusion sets in. Fatigue, hunger, overstimulation, or pain may all add to the unrest.

They're not being difficult. They're afraid, and often, they can't tell you why. Here's what you can do to add calm and direction.

- Turn on soft, warm lighting before sunset.
- Reduce loud background noise (TV, radios, even overlapping conversations).
- Light a lavender candle or diffuse calming essential oils.
- Sit near them. Your steady presence can ease their internal storm.
- Serve meals at consistent times, especially dinner.
- Avoid caffeine and sugar late in the day.
- Begin bedtime rituals early (folding a blanket, saying a prayer, humming a favorite tune).
- Familiar actions can soothe an unfamiliar mind.
- Don't argue when they insist it's time to leave. Instead, say something like, *"We'll head out soon. Let's rest for a moment first."*

- Offer comfort before correction. If they're angry, don't push back (step away, return gently).
- Match their emotional tone with compassion, not control.

Often, agitation is a signal vs. a symptom.

They may be:

- Hungry or thirsty
- Cold or in pain
- Needing the bathroom
- Scared by a shadow or startled by their reflection

This is where caregiving becomes soul work.

There may be evenings when you feel helpless, when their anger breaks your heart or their sadness makes you ache. You may feel like you've lost the person you once knew.

But remember this: *their spirit is still there.*

They may be hidden beneath the fog, but they are not gone. So hum the old songs. Rub their back. Say, *"I'm here. You're safe."* You are not failing. You are ministering at dusk.

Sundowning is not just a challenge.
It is a spiritual threshold.
It's a moment when your steady hands,
your quiet voice, your unwavering love
become the last anchor of the day.
So when the sun goes down,
don't just see confusion.
See a sacred call to presence.
Because even at dusk,
love can still shine through.

Chapter 14

CLOSING REFLECTION – THE JOURNEY OF LOVE & CARE

Caring for someone you love, whether it's a parent, spouse, sibling, or close friend, is one of the greatest acts of love a person can offer. It is not always easy, not always pretty, and certainly not always recognized. But it is holy work.

You are stepping into the role of comforter, advocate, protector, and presence. And that matters. Every quiet night, every repeated story, every wiped tear, every word of encouragement... it all matters.

If you've found this book, chances are you're in the thick of it or preparing to be. Maybe you're afraid. Maybe you're tired. Maybe you're just trying to figure out how to do the next right thing.

Let me say this: You are not alone.

Thousands of families are walking this road every single day. And while each journey is different, the heart behind it is the same—love. Love in action. Love that keeps showing up. Love that stays even when things get hard or confusing or sad.

This love is sacred. And it deserves to be nurtured, too.

You won't always get it right. You'll have days when your patience wears thin or when you feel like you've failed. You may second-guess yourself, feel overwhelmed, or wish you could do more.

Please know: Your presence is enough. Your care is enough.

No one can do this perfectly. And that's okay. What matters most is that you're trying, you're showing up, and you're doing it from a place of love. That is powerful. That is enough.

This book was never meant to give you every answer. It was meant to walk with you, to share pieces of wisdom from someone who has lived it, and to remind you that there is beauty in the caregiving journey.

Let it be a beginning:
- The beginning of a new level of understanding.
- The beginning of deeper compassion.
- The beginning of honoring both your loved one's life and your own.

May you walk this path with courage. May your hands be gentle, and your heart remain open. May you see the person behind the illness. May you find moments of laughter and grace.

May your love be felt deeply, daily, and without doubt. And when the road is long, may you remember: you are doing sacred work.

Appendix

CARE LOGS AND JOURNALS

Use this log to plan and track your loved one's daily care schedule.

Time	Activity / Notes
7:00 AM	
9:00 AM	
12:00 PM	
3:00 PM	
6:00 PM	
8:00 PM	

Use this journal page to record changes in behavior, mood, appetite, hygiene, or other observations. These notes can support communication with healthcare providers.

Date	Observation	Trigger	Resolution

Use this template to track a typical day for your loved one. Customize times and tasks as needed.

7:00 AM	Wake up / Personal hygiene
9:00 AM	Breakfast / Medications
12:00 PM	Lunch / Light exercise
3:00 PM	Snack / Music time
6:00 PM	Dinner / Conversation
8:00 PM	Prepare for bed / Soothing routine

Use this medication log to track your loved one's prescriptions, dosages, and times. This can help avoid missed or duplicated medications and assist during doctor visits.

Medication	Dosage	Time	Purpose	Given (✓)

ACKNOWLEDGEMENTS

Writing *From the Heart of a Caregiver* has been a labor of love, reflection, and deep gratitude. There are so many people who have walked beside me on this journey, through caregiving, storytelling, and soul work, and I want to take a moment to honor them.

First and foremost, I want to acknowledge God—my source, my strength, and my sustainer. It was His divine hand that placed every person, every opportunity, and even every challenge in my path for a greater purpose.

To my parents, Robert and Lydia, in loving memory—you gave me the foundation of love and family. That nurturing spirit you planted in me has grown into the work I've done for decades. I carry your values in every life I touch.

To my daughter, Kourtni Ayanna, and my granddaughter, Amiya—your unconditional love is a light in my life. You've shown me what love looks like in its purest, everyday form. You keep my heart full.

To my twin sister, Jacquelyn—thank you for always being a listening ear throughout the years. Your encouragement and understanding have meant the world to me. Though our gifts are expressed differently, yours with children and mine with the elderly—the heart of our work is the same: love, patience, and care. I see you; I honor you, and I love you deeply.

To my sister Asarene—you stepped in with love and grace and as our parents aged, you became our guide, advocate, and steady hand. You ushered Jacquelyn and me through life's milestones with quiet strength and care and I will forever be grateful.

To my siblings—Elvie, Verdene, and Robert and in loving memory of Freddie and Martha (Ann)—thank you for cheering me on, for being supportive, and for reminding me of the power of family unity.

To my sister/niece, Tracy—thank you for believing in my voice even before I did. You've pushed me gently but firmly to write this book, and I'm so grateful for your guidance, your heart, and your support. You rock, truly.

To my friend Mily—thank you for being a real friend, a soul friend who truly sees my heart and the work that I do. Thank you for being so encouraging and for honoring my calling every chance you get. Your support and love have uplifted me more than you know.

To Dulce—from the very beginning, you spoke life into me. Your encouraging words let me know that you saw me and the heart I put into my work. Thank you for always uplifting me and reminding me that what I do matters.

To Cheri—what a divine appointment it was when we met. You were looking for fellow caregivers for your client, and I was chosen. That moment sparked a beautiful and lasting friendship. Thank you for always being in my corner, for encouraging me, and for thinking of me for referrals. I'm so blessed that our paths crossed.

To Frank and Elissa, in loving memory—if I had to play favorites, it would be you. There was an unspoken bond that connected us from the start. You made me laugh, sometimes cry, but it was never a dull moment. You claimed me as your own and introduced me to others as your daughter, and I will forever hold that in my heart. Thank you to Frank and John for entrusting me to care for you. It was an honor.

And finally, to Mrs. Dugal, my high school writing and literature teacher—thank you for seeing something in me when I couldn't see it myself. You pulled the stories out of me when I thought I had nothing to say. This book was born in part because of you.

With love and gratitude,
Gwendolyn

About the Author

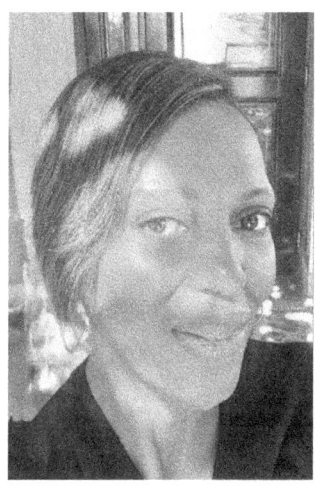

Gwendolyn Burrell is a Dallas-based caregiver, writer, and eldercare advocate with over twenty years of hands-on experience supporting seniors and their families. Her approach is rooted in compassion, dignity, and a deep belief in holistic healing that honors the physical, emotional, and spiritual needs of those in her care. A devoted caregiver, Gwendolyn has accompanied individuals through some of life's most tender and vulnerable moments, offering presence, clarity, and heartfelt guidance. She is especially passionate about preserving the humanity of those living with Alzheimer's and dementia, elevating the sacred role of caregivers, and helping families provide love-centered, respectful care. When she's not caring for others or writing, Gwendolyn finds joy in nature walks, herbal teas, and meaningful time with her family. *From the Heart of a Caregiver* is her debut book, a soulful offering to everyone navigating the caregiving journey.

www.ingramcontent.com/pod-product-compliance
Lightning Source LLC
Chambersburg PA
CBHW020604030426
42337CB00013B/1201